MY FEET ARE KILLIN' ME!

A Surgeon's Field Manual for Feet That Never Get a Day Off

Dr. James Whitfield

My Feet Are Killin' Me!

A Surgeon's Field Manual for Feet That Never Get a Day Off

Published by Melon Glow Books, an imprint of Melon Glow Company, LLC.

melonglowbooks.com

First Edition

ISBN: 979-8-9969954-9-3

Disclaimer

This book shares general information based on decades of clinical experience treating working professionals. It is not personalized medical advice and is not a substitute for evaluation by your own physician or podiatrist. If you have diabetes, poor circulation, neuropathy, or any condition affecting foot sensation or healing, consult a foot care professional before attempting any home care described here. Results vary by individual. If you experience redness, warmth, drainage, or pain at rest, seek professional care promptly.

Table of Contents

Chapter 1: On the Job with Feet Made of What?

> *Surgeon's Note: "Your shift doesn't end when you clock out; it ends when your feet stop screaming."*
>
> *If you are working a high-torque job, your foundation is the most critical piece of equipment you own.*

The first hour of your shift is a lie. You move with purpose, your stride is sharp, and the floor feels solid beneath you. You are the professional: the nurse heading to the station, the officer patrolling the beat, the waitress setting the tables. But somewhere around hour four, the lie unravels.

It starts as a subtle, low-frequency hum — a "slow creep." You aren't consciously thinking about your feet, but your body is already negotiating a truce with the ground. You stop heel-striking, shifting to a shuffling gait to minimize the impact. You adjust your weight, leaning slightly to the left to give the right arch a moment of respite. By hour eight, that hum has turned into a high-pitched buzz. Every step is no longer a movement; it is a negotiation with a surface that refuses to give, and every pulse of your heartbeat feels like it's hammering directly into the balls of your feet.

We call this "tired." We say, "My feet are killing me." But that is a surface-level diagnosis for a much deeper, structural failure.

I have often used the comparison of feet made of glass — the way a boxer can have a "glass jaw" —

because an abused foot can carry that same ultra-sensitivity, right up to sudden, total collapse. I've also made the comparison to "feet made of clay," which crumble, metaphorically speaking, like old dried-up clay after years of abuse. Here in this book, I'm throwing the kid gloves off, because I want your serious attention.

Your foundation — your feet — is made of muscle and bone supplied by blood vessels that are the longest pathway to travel from the heart. You are standing on concrete, wearing shoes that are essentially rigid, narrow coffins. With every shift of your weight, with every pivot at the terminal, with every step on a hard, unforgiving surface, you are creating microscopic fractures and bruises that accumulate daily. At first, they are invisible. You don't see them. You don't feel them — not until the end of the shift, when the "pittance of relief" you get from sitting down is suddenly not enough.

The Poor Relative

In the hierarchy of the human body, the foot is the furthest body part from the heart. Read that again.

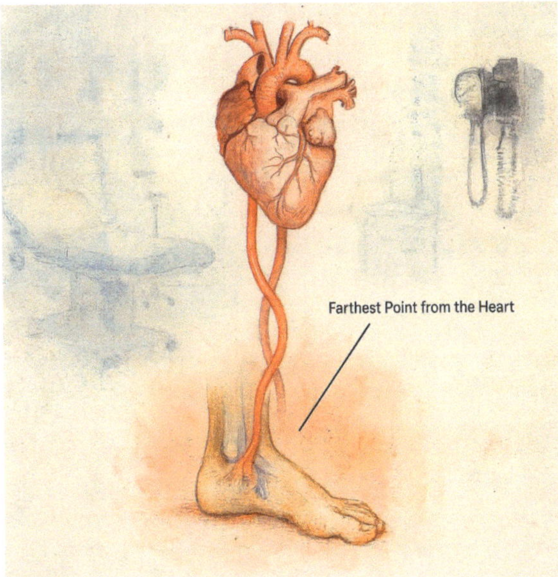

It is the distant relative we ignore until it begins to scream for attention. We spend our lives focusing on the mechanics of our hearts, our lungs, and our brains, while the foundation that bears every ounce of our burden is stuffed into restrictive, narrow "coffins" and forgotten.

This manual is a departure from that neglect. We are treating the foot not as a distant relative, but as the primary engine of your structural integrity. The following pages are not a textbook — they are a technical field manual designed to restore your foundation. We will identify the mechanical collapse caused by modern footwear, re-establish the Tripod, and execute a daily repair sequence to rebuild your stability from the ground up.

Your foundation is your future. Let's get to work.

The Energy Myth

You run on caffeine, tea, and the sheer necessity of getting through an eight-hour shift. You are the nurse in the ER, the officer on the beat, the waitress in the middle of a rush. You've tried every "fix" on the shelf: corn pads that slide, heel lifts that shift, and "coffin shoes" that pinch the life out of your stride. You know the irony: your body is exhausted, but the feet — the farthest point from your heart — receive only a pittance of the circulation and none of the energy-drink "lift" you keep pouring into your system.

This is the Energy Myth in action. We try to power our bodies like high-performance machines. We pour in the caffeine, we reach for the sugar, we rely on sheer professional grit to keep us upright. But we are fuel-starving the engine at its most critical point: the foundation. Your feet are the farthest point from your heart. Gravity is constantly pulling your blood away, and your rigid, "standard-issue" footwear acts as a tourniquet, preventing that life-sustaining circulation from reaching the very tissues taking the brunt of your professional life.

You are living in a state of chronic, metabolic debt. That burning sensation you feel at hour six? That isn't just pressure. That is a localized oxygen debt. Your feet are literally starving for the circulation your heart is trying to send — circulation your "coffin shoes" are blocking.

We have been conditioned to accept this. We wear the sleek leather, the stiff-soled trainers, the safety-toe boots that feel like iron boxes, all in the name of professional presentation. We believe that if a shoe doesn't "break in" — meaning, stretch your foot to fit the shoe's design — it isn't "quality." We are trading our long-term structural integrity for a momentary aesthetic.

But here is the truth the uniform suppliers won't tell you: You are not a victim of the shift. You are the architect of your own foundation.

The floor hasn't changed. The shoes haven't changed. But the way you understand the physics of standing is about to change. You are going to stop treating your feet as an afterthought and start treating them as the Tripod that holds your entire life upright.

In the chapters that follow, we are going to move from the problem — the crushing, suffocating reality of the Fragile Foot — to the solution. We are going to audit your gear, ritualize your recovery, and build a foundation that lasts for the next twenty years, not just the next twenty minutes.

You are done walking in coffins. From this point forward, you are going to walk on your own terms.

Chapter 2: The Tripod Principle

To fix the foundation, you must first understand the engineering of the foot. We have been sold a lie that the foot is a singular, monolithic block that simply "hits the ground." In reality, the foot is a sophisticated, three-point structural system.

When this system is balanced, you are a machine of efficiency. When it collapses, you are essentially a crumbling structure under load. I call this the Tripod Principle.

The Three Pillars of Stability

Your foot is built on three distinct points of contact. If one fails, the entire weight of your body — plus whatever gear, trays, or equipment you are carrying — is forced onto the remaining two. This is the moment of failure.

- **The Heel (The Anchor):** This is your base of operation. It is designed to take the initial impact of every step. When you stand still, your heel is the primary shock absorber for your spine. If your shoe restricts your heel or forces it to sit at an unnatural angle, you are effectively cutting your anchor chain. You'll feel the strain travel immediately up your Achilles into your calf.
- **The Big Toe Base (The Rudder):** This is the most critical point for propulsion and balance. Every time you shift to reach for a file, turn toward a patient, or pivot to serve a table, the Big Toe Base acts as your steering mechanism. If it is compressed into a narrow toe box, you lose your rudder. You become unstable, and

your body compensates by tightening the muscles in your shins and hips to keep you upright.

- **The Little Toe Base (The Stabilizer):** Often ignored, this point prevents you from tipping over. It provides the lateral stability required for every micro-adjustment you make while standing on uneven surfaces like tile, carpet, or concrete. When your shoe is too narrow, the Little Toe Base is crushed inward, causing the nerves between your toes to fire in protest — often resulting in that sharp, stinging pain that makes you want to rip your shoes off the moment you get to your car.

The Architecture of the Collapse

What happens when you stand for twelve hours in a coffin shoe?

Think of your Tripod as a stool. If you shorten one leg, the stool wobbles. If you compress all three legs inward, the stool buckles under the weight. When you force your foot into a narrow, rigid shoe, you are essentially pinning the three pillars of your Tripod together. You lose the natural "splay" — the way your foot is meant to widen and grip the floor as you put weight down.

When the Tripod cannot spread, the arch — the bridge connecting these three points — is forced to take all the tension. This is why "arch support" insoles are often just a band-aid. They are trying to hold up a bridge that has already lost its foundation.

Reclaiming the Geometry

You don't need fancy, high-tech insoles to fix this. You need geometry.

A healthy, functioning Tripod requires room. It needs a wide, flat platform that allows your Heel, Big Toe Base, and Little Toe Base to make firm contact with the floor independently. When these three points are engaged, the weight is distributed evenly. Your ankles stop wobbling, your knees stop locking, and your lower back stops absorbing the shock your feet were supposed to handle.

In the next chapter, we will look at exactly how we've been tricked into buying "coffin shoes" that systematically dismantle this Tripod, and how to spot them before they ever make it into your closet.

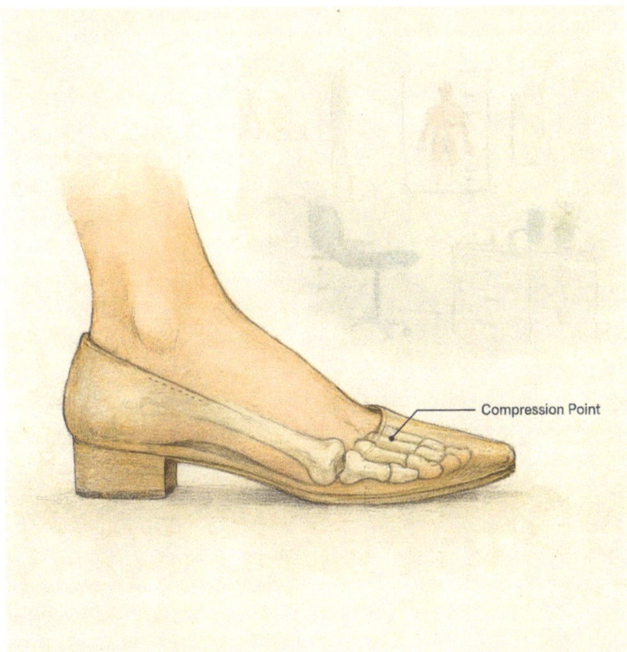

> *Illustrator's Note: A top-down, x-ray style view of a foot with three glowing points highlighting the*

> *Heel, Big Toe Base, and Little Toe Base, connected by a triangular web. Beneath it, two side-by-side icons: a wide, balanced Stable Tripod, and a squeezed, distorted Collapsed Tripod representing the coffin effect.*

Chapter 3: The Coffin Shoe

We have established the Tripod — the Heel, the Big Toe Base, and the Little Toe Base. It is a masterpiece of biological engineering, designed to bear your weight and guide your movement. So why, when you walk into a store to buy work shoes, are you presented with footwear that seems designed to dismantle that very architecture?

Welcome to the Coffin Shoe.

The Aesthetics Trap

The problem begins with a fundamental misunderstanding of what a "professional" shoe looks like. For decades, the industry has equated "professional" with "streamlined." Think of the classic black leather lace-up, the sleek stewardess pump, or the modern, lightweight trainer. They are narrow at the front, tapered at the toes, and often feature a raised heel or a rigid, stiff sole.

From an aesthetic standpoint, these shoes are beautiful. They fit the uniform. They look clean, polished, and sharp. But from a biomechanical standpoint, they are functional disasters. They force your toes into a cramped, unnatural position, effectively pinning your Big Toe Base and Little Toe Base together.

When you pin the pillars of your Tripod, you aren't walking; you are balancing on a block.

The "Break-In" Lie

The most dangerous piece of advice you will ever receive in a shoe store is: "Don't worry, they'll break in."

Let's be clear: your feet should not be the ones doing the breaking. If a shoe is so rigid that it requires your foot to stretch the leather or mold the synthetic materials through sheer force of will, you are wearing a Coffin. By the time that shoe "breaks in," it has already forced your bones into a compromised position, likely creating the very bunions, hammertoes, and nerve compressions you are trying to avoid.

A quality shoe should fit your foot the moment you slide it on. If it doesn't, it doesn't matter how professional it looks — it is not for you.

The Anatomy of the Coffin

How do you spot a Coffin Shoe before you buy it? Look for these three fatal flaws:

- **The Tapered Toe:** Look at the shoe from above. If it doesn't have a wide, square-ish, or rounded front that mimics the natural splay of your toes, it is a Coffin.
- **The Rigid Sole:** Try to bend the shoe. If you can't bend it easily at the ball of the foot — where your toes naturally flex — it is a Coffin.
- **The "Drop" Heel:** Look at the shoe from the side. If the heel is significantly higher than the forefoot, even slightly, it shifts your center of gravity forward, jamming your toes into the front of the shoe.

It is time to stop buying into the "standard issue" and start buying for your survival. In the next chapter, we will walk through the Professional Profiles, where we see exactly how these Coffin Shoes manifest in the specific, daily grinds of the nurse, the officer, the waitress, and the stewardess.

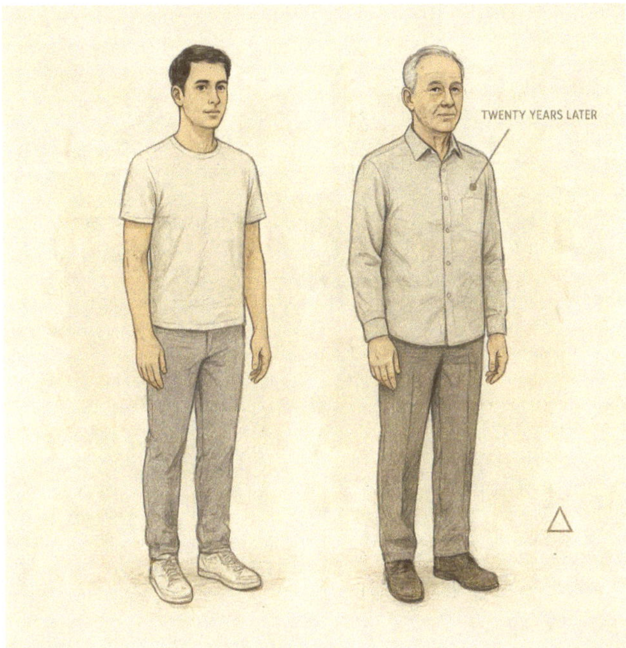

> *Illustrator's Note: A ghosted x-ray view of a foot inside a sleek, polished professional shoe, showing the bones of the toes squeezed into a sharp point, overlaid with a faint red outline of a wide, natural, splayed foot to visualize the tourniquet effect.*

Chapter 4: Professional Profiles — The Frontline Reality

The "Glass Foot" doesn't discriminate based on your industry, but it attacks in different ways depending on your movement patterns. To understand how to heal, we must first recognize how we break. Let's look at how the Tripod fails in four of our most demanding, high-stakes professions.

The Nurse's Pivot: The Static Trap

The hospital floor is an unforgiving landscape of industrial tile — a surface that absorbs nothing and reflects every ounce of impact back into your joints. For a nurse, the danger isn't just distance; it's the static-to-dynamic transition.

You spend forty minutes standing perfectly still at a terminal, documenting, before suddenly needing to pivot 180 degrees and dash down the hall to a room. In that moment of the "Pivot," your Big Toe Base is meant to be your rudder. But in a tapered, stiff-soled nursing clog, you can't splay. Your foot acts like a block of wood. To compensate, your ankle muscles tighten, and you "shear" across the floor rather than gripping it. By hour six, that pivot becomes a source of agony.

> *Nurse's Field Note: The next time you're at the terminal, don't just stand. If you find yourself locking your knees, you've already lost your Tripod. Practice the Arch Lift — a micro-contraction of your foot muscles — to keep the foundation awake while you type.*

The Officer's Burden: The Armor Load

If the nurse is defined by the pivot, the police officer is defined by the Load. You are carrying a belt weighted down with gear, body armor, and tech. Your center of gravity is constantly being pulled and shifted.

Because you are carrying extra weight, your Heel — the anchor — is under constant, heavy pressure. If your patrol boots have a raised heel, your body is effectively being pushed into a perpetual state of forward fall. By the end of a shift, your boots feel like concrete blocks, and you feel the buzzing in your Little Toe Base from fighting to stabilize that gear-load on uneven surfaces.

> *Officer's Field Note: Your boots are the most important piece of tactical gear you own. If they don't allow your toes to splay under the weight of your kit, you are not "tactically prepared" — you are walking on a ticking time bomb of structural failure.*

The Waitress's Endurance: The "Mile-Marker" Fatigue

In a restaurant, the floor is your office, and it is almost always hard, unforgiving tile. You are trapped in a cycle of carry-and-turn, navigating tight spaces, balancing trays, and constantly decelerating to stop at tables. Every time you stop, you brake with your Little Toe Base. In thin-soled or "non-slip" shoes lacking a proper Tripod base, that braking force has nowhere to go — it travels straight up into your knees and hips.

> *Waitress's Field Note: You are an endurance athlete who doesn't get to wear running shoes. Treat your non-slips like precision equipment. If they don't have a stable, anatomical platform, you are essentially serving tables on stilts.*

The Stewardess's Stance: The "Galley-Squeeze"

Flight attendants face a unique set of constraints: narrow aisles, confined spaces, and pressure to maintain a specific, often restrictive, aesthetic. You are rarely walking long distances; you are stationed in confined areas, standing on surfaces that vibrate with the aircraft's engines. The "Galley-Squeeze" crushes your Little Toe Base and keeps your Heel under constant tension. The fatigue here is vascular — blood pools in your feet, causing that heavy, lead-like sensation that doesn't go away even after you kick your shoes off in the hotel room.

> *Stewardess's Field Note: The Galley-Squeeze is a trap. Even in two square feet of space, you can perform a Weight Shift. If you are standing, move. If you are leaning, switch sides. Never let your foundation go completely static.*

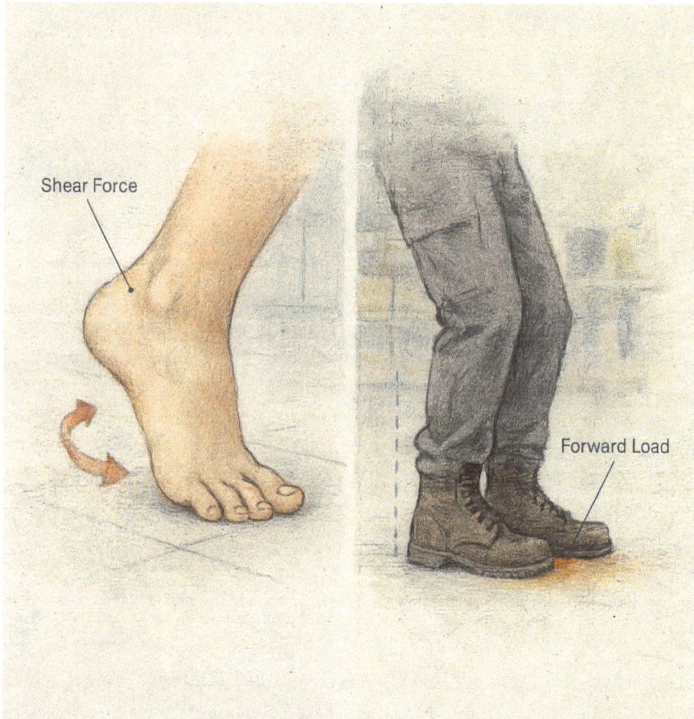

Bridging to the Toolkit

We've seen the Nurse, the Officer, the Waitress, and the Stewardess. Their environments differ — the hospital, the street, the restaurant, the aircraft — but the culprit is identical. They are all battling the Fragile Foot caused by the same mechanical failure: the loss of the Tripod.

They have all been misled by the Energy Myth, believing the solution is to power through the pain, when in reality they are simply waiting for the inevitable day their foundation finally cracks.

But the pattern is now broken. Because they — and you — now understand why the collapse happens, we can move from the Why to the How. Before we get to the Toolkit, though, there's one specific piece of wreckage we need to look at directly: what all those years in a Coffin Shoe can actually leave behind on your toes.

Chapter 5: The Wreckage Report — Hammer Toes and the Corns They Leave Behind

> *Surgeon's Note: A corn is not bad luck. It is a receipt. Your shoe has been billing your toe for years, and the skin finally started keeping a paper trail.*
>
> *If your Tripod has been living in a Coffin Shoe long enough, eventually the Coffin leaves a signature.*

Not every professional who reads this book will develop a hammer toe. But if you've spent a decade or two standing on concrete and tile in a shoe that tapers to a point, there's a real chance you already have one — or you're watching one form right now, and you've been calling it something else. "My toe's just a little crooked." "I've got a rough spot that won't go away." "It's just a callus, everybody gets those."

I've spent over thirty years hearing "my feet are killin' me" walk through the door in exactly this shape. So let's call it what it is, and then let's talk about what you can actually do about it — starting today, whether or not you ever set foot in a surgeon's office.

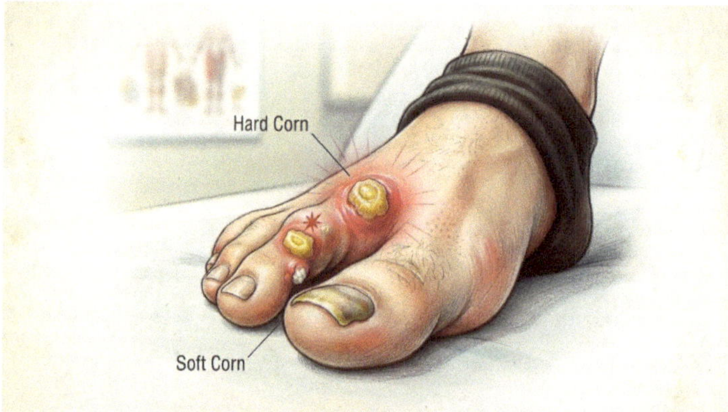

How the Coffin Writes Its Signature

Remember the Tripod: the Heel, the Big Toe Base, and the Little Toe Base. When a shoe tapers and pins those pillars together for eight, ten, twelve hours a day, something has to give. Usually it's the second toe. The middle joint starts riding up, the tip starts pointing down, and the muscles on top of the toe tighten while the ones underneath go slack and weak. Early on, the joint is still flexible — you can push it back down with your finger. Give it long enough in the Coffin, and it stiffens into that position permanently. That's a hammer toe.

The corn on top isn't a separate problem. It's your skin doing exactly what skin is built to do: thickening up wherever a bent knuckle keeps grinding against the roof of a shoe. The trouble is that the thickened skin then becomes part of the injury. It takes up more room in a space that was already too tight, and it presses straight down on the nerve endings underneath. Patients have described it to me the same way for three decades: “It feels like there's a pebble under my toe and I keep checking my shoe for something that isn't there.”

None of this happened because you did something wrong. It happened because your shoes have been narrower than your foot for longer than your foot could tolerate. It's mechanics, not fate.

What It Actually Steals

This rarely shows up as one dramatic injury. It shows up as a slow shrinking of what you're willing to do. "I can only wear these two pairs of shoes now. Everything else hurts within an hour." "I don't take my shoes off at the beach anymore." "My knee started hurting because I've been walking funny to keep weight off that toe — now I've got two problems instead of one."

That last one matters for you especially, because you're already asking your knees, hips, and low back to absorb a full shift's worth of compensation for a Tripod that isn't landing evenly. A hammer toe doesn't just hurt where it lives. It changes your entire gait, and the bill gets forwarded up the chain.

Handling It Today — Safe Home Care

You don't need to wait for a diagnosis to start taking pressure off. A few cautions first: if you have diabetes, poor circulation, neuropathy, or notably thin skin, don't self-treat aggressively — have a podiatrist handle any trimming. If the area is ever red, hot, oozing, or painful even at rest, that's a same-week appointment, not a home project.

For everyone else, here's the routine that actually holds up over time:

- **Soak to soften.** Ten to fifteen minutes in warm water, a couple times a week. Dry thoroughly afterward.
- **File gently, never cut.** A pumice stone or emery board while the skin is soft. Take a little at a time. No blades, no scissors, no "bathroom surgery." Stop if you see pink.
- **Urea cream, daily.** A 10–40% urea cream softens the thickened skin between filings without the harshness of acid-based corn removers, which can burn healthy skin around the corn.
- **Offload, don't just cushion.** A donut pad, moleskin, or gel toe sleeve placed around the corn — not on top of it — takes the shoe's pressure off the exact spot that's screaming.
- **Fix the shoe.** Everything above buys you comfort. Only a wider, deeper toe box (see the Shoe Audit) stops the corn from simply reforming, since the mechanical cause never left.

Waking the Muscles Back Up

Pads and creams treat the symptom. These small daily moves work the actual imbalance — the tight top-of-toe tendons and the weak little muscles that are supposed to hold the toe flat:

- **Toe spreads:** Spread all your toes apart as wide as you can, hold, release. Ten to fifteen reps.
- **The Short Foot exercise:** Without curling your toes, draw the ball of your foot toward your heel, like gently shortening your own arch. Hold five to ten seconds. This is the single best

exercise for waking up the small stabilizer muscles of the Tripod.

- **Towel scrunches:** Toes only, scrunch a towel toward you across the floor. Ten to twenty reps.

Do these barefoot, five to ten minutes, once or twice a day. Nobody straightens a toe in a week. Patients who stuck with it for four to eight weeks were the ones who noticed the corn had stopped getting worse and the ache had eased — not because the toe went perfectly straight, but because the pressure driving it finally dropped.

When the Toe Won't Budge Anymore

If you try to push the toe straight with your own finger while sitting down and it simply won't move, you're past the flexible stage. That doesn't mean surgery is your only remaining option — it means the goal shifts from straighten it to stop it from getting worse and take the pain down. Buddy-taping the toe to its neighbor with a bit of padding between them, a gel or spring-loaded toe splint worn at night, extra-depth shoes with a shoe-stretcher applied exactly at the pressure point, and regular professional trimming can carry a genuinely rigid toe for years without an operation. One patient in her late sixties put it best: "It's not straight, but I can shop for an hour now without crying on the way home."

If, after a real effort over several months, you're still dealing with constant pain, skin breakdown that won't heal, or a quality of life that's genuinely collapsing — that's the point to have an honest surgical conversation with a podiatrist, on your terms, not out of desperation.

Field Note: A corn is a pressure gauge, not a life sentence. Read it, relieve it, and keep your Tripod on the case. Most of the damage is reversible if you stop feeding it.

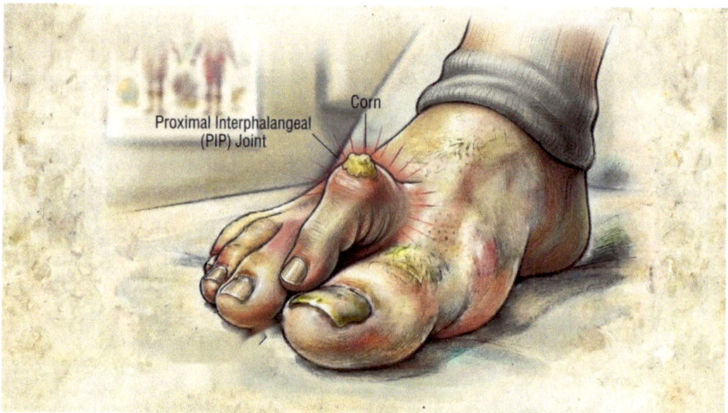

Illustrator's Note: Two side-by-side line illustrations. Panel A: a healthy Tripod with the second toe lying flat, the triangular platform intact. Panel B: the same foot in cross-section inside a tapered Coffin Shoe, the second toe buckled upward at the middle joint, a small red pressure zone marking where the corn is forming. Caption: "Same foot. Different shoe. Ten years apart."

Chapter 6: The Daily Inspection Ritual

If you owned a high-performance vehicle, you wouldn't just drive it until the wheels fell off and then wonder why it stopped moving. You would check the tire pressure, the oil, and the alignment. Your feet are the tires of your professional life, and yet most of us only pay attention to them when they are screaming in pain.

The Daily Inspection Ritual is the moment you transition from a passive victim of the Glass Foot to the primary maintainer of your foundation. It takes exactly two minutes, requires no special equipment, and can be done the moment you walk through your front door.

The Three-Step Scan

When you get home and remove your Coffin Shoes, do not just throw them in the closet and collapse. Sit down, take a breath, and perform this scan.

- **The Temperature Check:** Feel your feet with your hands. Are they unnaturally hot? Heat is the universal language of inflammation — your body telling you the circulatory tax has been paid in full.
- **The Red-Zone Audit:** Look for red marks, calluses, or swelling, specifically on the outside of the Little Toe Base and the top of the Big Toe Base. These are your pressure maps. If you see these marks daily, your shoes are officially unfit for duty.
- **The Splay Test:** Place your bare foot on the floor. Do your toes naturally spread, or do they

remain cramped in the shape of your shoe? If they stay curled even after you've taken your shoes off, you're experiencing neuromuscular lock — your feet have forgotten how to be feet.

The Recovery Protocol

Once you've identified the stress, perform these three quick actions to reset the system:

- **Elevate:** Prop your feet up above the level of your heart for 5 minutes to drain pooled fluid.
- **Toe Release:** Use your hands to manually spread your toes apart and massage the skin between them, breaking the tension the coffin created during the day.
- **The Ball-Roll:** Roll the arch of your foot over a tennis ball or frozen water bottle for 60 seconds per foot to desensitize nerves under constant pressure.

Most professionals experience the Glass Foot as a slow, accumulating injury. They don't have a bad day that ruins their feet; they have six years of bad days that lead to chronic, career-ending pain. By performing this ritual, you are effectively resetting the clock — you are performing preventative maintenance, not just relaxing after work.

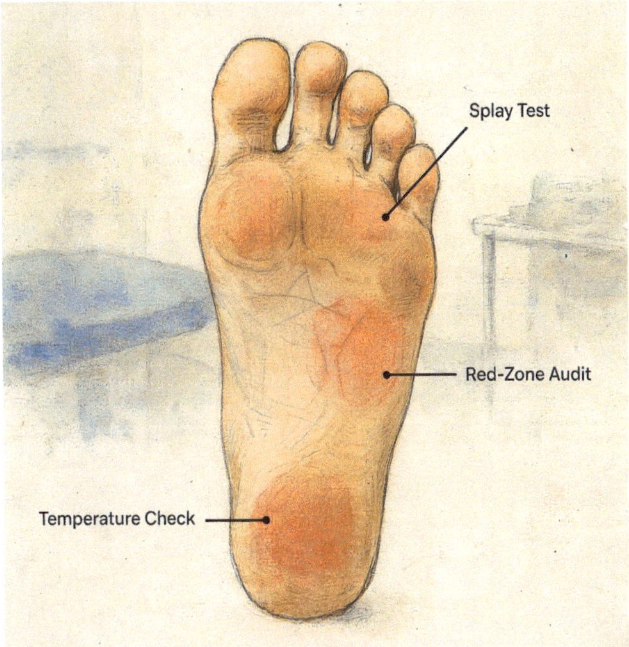

Illustrator's Note: An illustration of a foot with Hot Zones highlighted in red (heel, ball of foot, sides of toes), with a legend: Red Heat = Inflammation (Elevate). Red Marks = Pressure (Need a wider shoe). Curled Toes = Fatigue (Perform toe-spreads).

Chapter 7: The Shoe Audit

You now know how to inspect your feet. But if you walk into your next shift wearing the same Coffin Shoes you wore today, you are just mopping up water in a room with a leaky ceiling. It is time to stop the leak.

This is the Shoe Audit. You don't need a degree in biomechanics to do this; you just need to stop trusting the marketing on the box and start trusting the geometry of your own anatomy.

The Three-Minute Audit

- **The Splay Test (Width):** Remove the insole from your shoe, place it on the floor, and stand on it with your full body weight. If your foot hangs over the edges, your foot is wider than the shoe's internal chamber. That isn't a snug fit — it's a structural prison.
- **The Flex-Point Test (Flexibility):** Hold the shoe by the heel and toe and try to bend it in half. A healthy shoe bends only at the ball of the foot, exactly where your toes flex. If it's stiff as a board or bends in the arch, it's fighting your mechanics.
- **The Drop Test (Neutrality):** Place the shoe on a flat surface and look at it from the side. If the heel sits significantly higher than the front, even a small drop forces your weight onto your Big Toe Base. Look for a Zero-Drop or neutral sole.

The Anti-Coffin Shopping Checklist

- **Wide Toe Box:** A rounded or squared-off front. Your toes should never touch the sides of the shoe.
- **Thin, Flexible Sole:** Ground feel is sensory data your brain uses to stabilize your body.
- **Secure Midfoot:** Loose at the toes, but secure and firm across the midfoot and heel.
- **Breathable/Non-Binding Material:** Avoid stiff, heavy leathers that don't move.

A Note on Transitioning: if you've been wearing Coffin Shoes for ten years, your feet have likely lost some natural strength. Don't throw your old shoes away and run a marathon in minimalist footwear tomorrow. Start by wearing your new, anatomical Cradle shoes for the first four hours of your shift, then switch back if you feel extreme fatigue. Over two weeks, increase the time in your new shoes. You are building a new foundation; do it with patience, not speed.

Caution: this is not a guide for Birkenstocks, flip-flops, or lightweight lifestyle footwear. Those options lack the lateral support required for high-stakes, professional pivots and heavy gear loads. You are looking for Work-Oriented Anatomical Footwear — shoes that meet the same safety and durability requirements as your current uniform, but with an anatomical geometry that prevents the Glass Foot collapse.

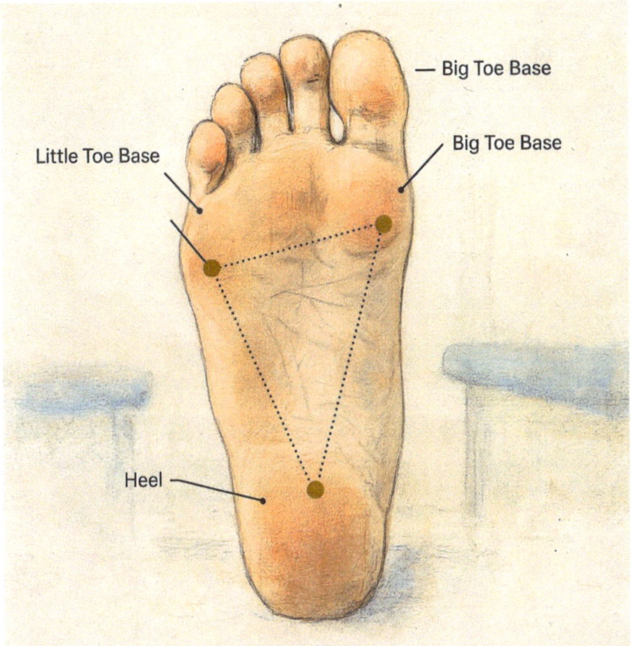

Illustrator's Note: Panel A — a foot standing on a Coffin insole, outer edges shaded red to show pressure overhang. Panel B — a foot on an Anatomical insole, contained perfectly within the lines. Caption: "Your foot should never be wider than the floor it stands on."

Chapter 8: Tactical Relief — The 4-Hour Rescue

You've performed your audit, you've picked your Cradle shoes, and you're back on the clock. But you're still working a long shift, and physics doesn't stop just because you bought better gear. The Glass Foot is a cumulative problem — the longer you stand, the more your foundation fatigues.

This is where Tactical Relief comes in. These are Micro-Resets you can perform in seconds, right in the middle of your shift, without leaving the floor.

The Gravity-Dump (15 Seconds)

Whenever you find 15 seconds of stillness, shift your weight entirely onto one leg. Lift the other foot slightly and wiggle your toes. This tells your brain your feet aren't trapped, and gives the compressed tissues in your arch a chance to re-inflate with blood. Switch legs and repeat.

The Calf-Pump (10 Reps)

Rise up onto your toes slowly, engage your calf muscles, then lower your heels back down. Ten reps. You are literally pumping the pooled fluid out of your feet and back into circulation — the ultimate antidote to the heavy, lead-like sensation.

The Arch-Grip (Hold for 5 Seconds)

While standing flat, imagine shortening your foot by pulling the Big Toe Base toward your Heel without curling your toes. Hold this grip for 5 seconds. You'll feel the tiny muscles in your arch engage, waking up the Tripod and taking weight off your ligaments.

These aren't stretches — they are tactical interruptions. If you feel the buzz start in your Little Toe Base, do a Calf-Pump. If you feel the heat rising in your arch, do a Gravity-Dump. You are not waiting for pain to tell you when to move; you are moving to prevent the pain from ever starting.

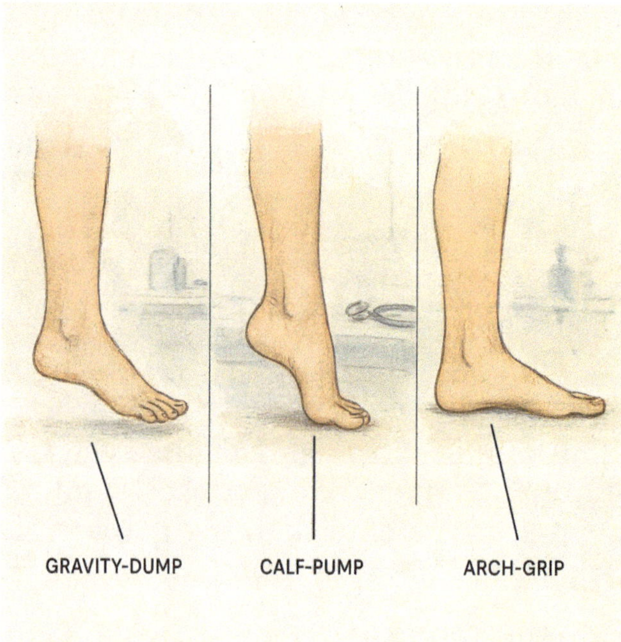

> *Illustrator's Note: A pocket-sized Rescue Card graphic with a simple flow chart: Feel Heat? → Gravity Dump. Feel Heavy? → Calf-Pump. Feel Collapse? → Arch-Grip. Operator-style clean lines, like a piece of gear that belongs in a uniform pocket.*

Chapter 9: Mapping Your Load — The Shift-Pressure Diary

You are now a tactical operator of your own foundation. You've audited your gear and learned the rescue techniques. But there is one final piece of the puzzle: Data.

Most people think their foot pain is a mysterious, unpredictable enemy. They blame it on "a long day" or "bad luck." But your pain is actually a data trail. If you can track when, where, and why your foundation fails, you can move from reacting to pain to anticipating it. Welcome to the Shift-Pressure Diary.

The Science of the Load

Pain is not a signal that you have failed; it is a signal that your Load has exceeded your Capacity. Your Load is composed of three variables: the Environment (concrete, tile, or carpet; flat or inclined), the Movement (static or dynamic), and the Duration (hours since your last Micro-Reset).

The Diary Framework

You don't need a complex system. A simple notebook or note-app will do. At the end of every shift, or during your mid-shift break, log these four markers:

Time	Surface	Intensity (1-10)	Relief Action Taken
Hr 2	Tile (Static)	2	None
Hr 5	Asphalt (Load)	6	10 Calf-Pumps
Hr 8	Concrete	8	Gravity-Dump

Decoding the Patterns

- **The Surface Spike:** If pain always spikes at the 4-hour mark regardless of what you do, your current shoes are likely failing on that surface.
- **The Static Stall:** If pain only spikes after standing still for over an hour, your issue is circulatory — increase your Tactical Relief frequency.
- **The Load Warning:** If pain increases on days you carry extra equipment, you've identified a weight-capacity issue — focus on strengthening the Arch-Grip.

The Diary turns your body into an experiment. When you show up to work, you aren't just showing up — you are a professional who knows exactly how much load your foundation can carry and exactly how to reset it before it hits the breaking point.

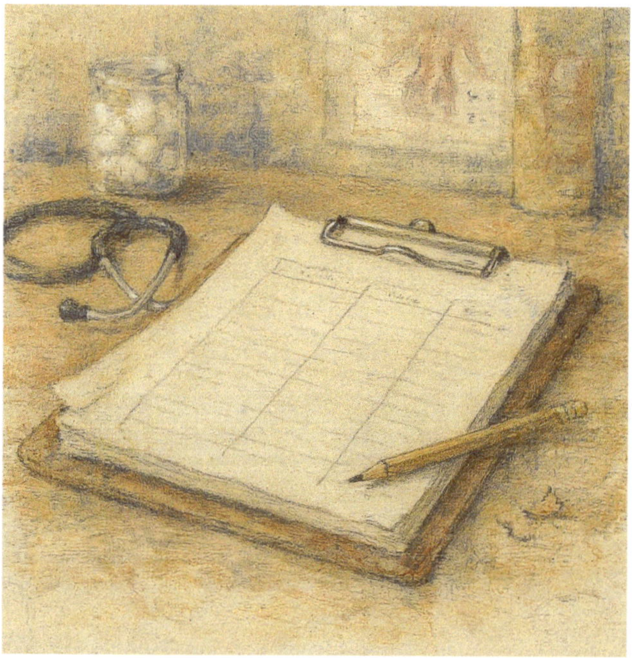

> *Illustrator's Note: A clean, black-and-white tactical log layout. Caption: "Do not be lazy with the data. A blank log is a missed opportunity to outsmart your pain."*

Chapter 10: Mastering the Micro-Break — The Science of Recovery

We have discussed the Tactical Relief techniques, but mastering the Micro-Break is not just about the how — it is about the when and the mindset.

In the high-pressure world of professional work, taking a break is often viewed as a weakness. We are conditioned to push through. The Micro-Break is the antidote to that cultural trap — a radical act of self-preservation that takes place in plain sight.

The Hidden Rhythm

The greatest mistake professionals make is waiting for their feet to scream “Stop!” before resting. By then, the inflammation has already set in. The Micro-Break is designed to be preemptive. Train your brain to recognize the sub-threshold signals: the Weight-Shift Urge (that subconscious feeling of wanting to lean or cross your ankles — execute a Gravity-Dump), and the Terminal Buzz (numbness or pins and needles — perform a Calf-Pump).

The Art of the Invisible Reset

- **The Listen-and-Release:** While standing in a static trap during a briefing or conversation, unlock your knees and shift 80% of your weight to your right foot, switching sides every 30 seconds. To an observer, you're just engaged. To your foundation, you're cycling load and rest.
- **The Counter-Lever:** If working at a counter, lean into it slightly, taking 5–10% of your body weight off your feet.

- **The Active Splay:** Mentally scan your toes throughout your shift. Are they curled or jammed together? Consciously spread them. If you can't, your shoe is too tight.

Exhaustion is not a linear function of time; it is a function of metabolic stagnation. Every Micro-Break acts as a valve, releasing pressure and allowing fresh, oxygenated blood back to the tissue. By the end of your shift, you won't just be less tired — you'll have a surplus of energy because you didn't spend the day fighting your own structural collapse.

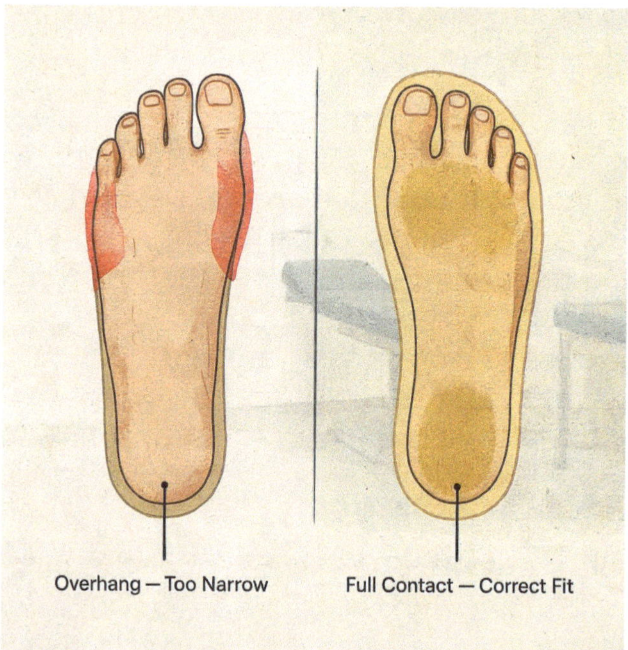

> *Illustrator's Note: Split-frames showing a professional in the same environment. Frame A (The Trap): rigid, locked posture. Frame B (The Reset): the same professional with subtle arrows showing weight shifting side to side, knees slightly bent, looking natural but actively engaged.*

Chapter 11: The Rebuilding Phase

You have the tools, the tactical mindset, and the data-tracking diary. You are ready to switch your gear and revolutionize your daily movement. But there is a final, critical hurdle: The Transition.

Many people fail here because they treat their feet like a light switch — flipping from Coffin Shoes to Anatomical Cradles in a single day. This is a mistake. Your feet have spent years adapting to the artificial support and restrictive shape of your old footwear. If you rush this transition, you won't just get sore; you'll trigger an inflammatory response. Do not let that happen.

The Two-Week Wake-Up Protocol

- **Days 1-3: The Split-Shift Rule.** Wear your new Cradle shoes for the first two to three hours of your shift only, then switch back to your old shoes for the remainder.
- **Days 4-7: The Active Hours Extension.** Add one hour of Cradle time each day, staying diligent about your Tactical Relief.
- **Days 8-14: The Full-Shift Calibration.** By the end of week two, you should be in your Cradle shoes for the full shift. If you still feel significant pain, review your Shift-Pressure Diary.

Managing the New Discomfort

You need to distinguish between Good Tired and Bad Hurt. Good Tired feels like a light, dull ache in the arches — the same feeling you get in your biceps after a good workout. It means your muscles are finally taking the load. Bad Hurt is sharp, stabbing, or hot. If you feel this, back off, take a day in your old shoes, and restart the Split-Shift protocol. You are building a foundation for the next twenty years; there is no prize for doing it in twenty days.

As you transition, pay attention to the floor. You will notice the texture of the tile, the temperature of the concrete, the subtle vibration of the building — this is Proprioception, your brain's ability to see the ground through your feet. By the time you finish these two weeks, the Glass Foot will no longer be your reality. You are no longer breaking in a shoe; you are building up a foundation.

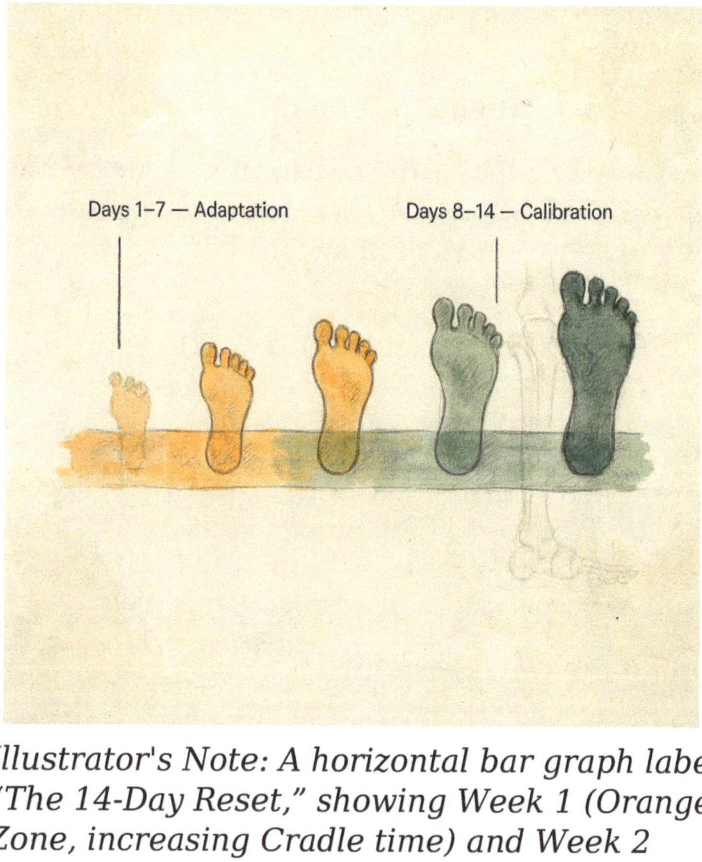

> *Illustrator's Note: A horizontal bar graph labeled "The 14-Day Reset," showing Week 1 (Orange Zone, increasing Cradle time) and Week 2 (Green Zone, full-shift wear), with a Foot-*

> *Strength icon that grows in intensity as days progress.*

Chapter 12: The Long Game — Protecting the Foundation

You have reached the end of the transition. Your Glass Foot is a memory, your Coffin Shoes are collecting dust, and you have built a foundation that works for you, not against you.

But here is the final truth: the shift never ends. The floor remains hard, the hours remain long, and the professional pressure to power through will always be there. If you stop maintaining your foundation, it will slowly revert. This final chapter is about shifting from Recovery to Sustainment.

The Quarterly Audit

Your feet are dynamic, but so is your work environment. Every three months, pull out your Shift-Pressure Diary and spend one week logging your data again. Are pain levels creeping up? Is there a new hot spot forming? Use this data to adjust your footwear or routine before the pain becomes chronic.

The Off-Duty Rebellion

Many professionals spend their work life in restrictive shoes, then spend their weekend in even more restrictive dress shoes or high-end fashion sneakers. Give your feet freedom time. Go barefoot whenever safely possible at home. Walk on grass or sand. These surfaces provide the sensory feedback your feet crave and force the small muscles of your Tripod to work in ways they can't on flat, predictable tile.

The Foundation First Mentality

You are now a different kind of professional. When you see a colleague limping at the end of a shift, complaining about their back, or reaching for painkillers, you now see the Glass Foot in them. Share the Tripod Principle. Tell them about the Coffin Shoe. By helping others fix their foundation, you reinforce your own commitment to the long game.

The Goal: Twenty Years of Ease

The goal of this book was never to just get you through the next shift. It was to ensure you are still standing, still moving, and still capable of doing the work you love twenty years from now.

You have traded the Energy Myth — the lie that you can power through structural collapse — for the Architecture of Stability. You are no longer a victim of the environment. You are the architect of your own performance. You don't just stand; you inhabit the ground. You don't just walk; you navigate the shift.

You are finished with the Glass Foot. Step forward.

Conclusion: You are the primary maintainer of your foundation. You don't just stand; you navigate the shift. This isn't just about tomorrow — it's about your ability to perform your job for the years until you retire with that pension. You are protecting a career.

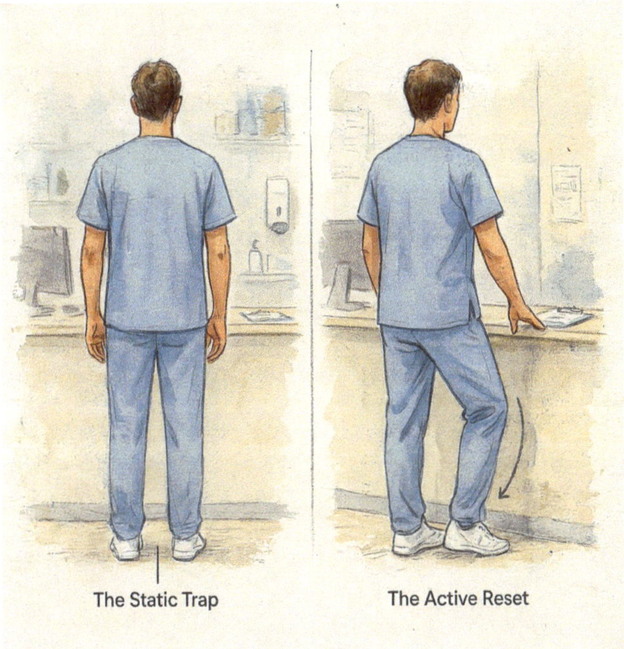

Illustrator's Note: An inspiring image of a professional at the start of their career, followed by the same professional twenty years later, standing with the same balanced, strong posture. Caption: "A foundation built on physics lasts a career. A foundation built on grit lasts until it breaks." A small tripod symbol on the closing page.

Appendix: The Professional's Field Manual

This section is designed to be your quick-reference guide during your shift. Keep this page bookmarked or printed as a pocket card.

1. The Daily Inspection Checklist

- **Temperature Check:** Feel for radiating heat. (If yes: Elevate.)
- **Red-Zone Audit:** Check for pressure points. (If yes: Widen your footwear.)
- **Splay Test:** Are toes cramped? (If yes: Perform Toe-Releases.)

2. The Tactical Relief Cheat Sheet

- **For Heavy/Lead Legs (Calf-Pump):** 10 repetitions, slow rise and fall.
- **For Hot/Inflamed Feet (Gravity-Dump):** 15 seconds per leg, wiggle toes.
- **For Collapsed Arches (Arch-Grip):** 5-second isometric hold, no toe curling.

3. The 14-Day Transition Log

A structured, two-week wake-up protocol that helps your feet safely adapt to new anatomical Cradle footwear without triggering an inflammatory response.

- **Days 1-3:** Split-shift — wear your new shoes for the first two to three hours before switching back to your old footwear.

- **Days 4–7:** Add one hour of wear time to your new shoes each day.
- **Days 8–14:** Full-shift calibration — move into your new shoes for the entirety of your workday.

Throughout this period, distinguish between Good Tired (a dull ache in the arches) and Bad Hurt (sharp, stabbing, or hot pain). If you experience Bad Hurt, back off and restart the protocol.

4. The Professional "Cradle" Criteria

This is not a guide for Birkenstocks, flip-flops, or lightweight lifestyle footwear — those lack the lateral stability needed for the Nurse's Pivot or the Officer's Burden. Here is how to define genuine Work-Oriented Anatomical Footwear:

- **Structural Integrity:** A firm midfoot and heel cup that stabilizes the foot for standing, pivoting, and walking on industrial surfaces without the shoe folding or losing shape.
- **Geometric Volume:** A wide, square, or rounded toe box that allows the Big Toe and Little Toe to maintain the Tripod base even after hours on your feet.
- **Zero-Drop Sole:** A level sole, heel not elevated above the forefoot, preventing the forward-fall sensation that overloads your arches.
- **Professional Pivot Stability:** A high-traction, secure outsole that allows rapid, controlled directional changes without the shoe sliding around the foot.

- **Structured Midfoot Containment:** A firm, secure lacing or closure system that locks the midfoot down during high-intensity shifts.
- **Industrial-Grade, Responsive Materials:** Durable, wear-resistant, and breathable enough to let the foot's intrinsic muscles move and work naturally.

The Foot Type Self-Assessment — The Wet Footprint Test

Before you go shopping for Cradle footwear, it helps to know exactly what kind of foot you're building for. This takes two minutes and no special equipment.

How to run the test

- **Step 1:** Wet the sole of your bare foot — a damp towel works fine.
- **Step 2:** Step firmly, once, onto a paper grocery bag, a piece of cardboard, or a dry section of pavement or garage floor. Keep your weight even, the way you'd stand naturally.
- **Step 3:** Step off and look at the shape you left behind.

Reading your print

- **Flat / Low Arch:** You see almost the entire sole, with a wide, solid connection between the heel and the forefoot. Little to no curve on the inside edge.
- **Neutral Arch:** You see a moderate curve on the inside edge — roughly half of the middle of the foot is visible, half is not.
- **High Arch:** You see only a thin sliver connecting the heel and forefoot, or the print looks like it's missing the middle section almost entirely.

What your type means for your Cradle shoe

- **Flat / Low Arch:** Prioritize a shoe with strong midfoot containment (Chapter 7) — your Tripod needs a firmer platform to keep from over-splaying under load.

- **Neutral Arch:** The standard Cradle Criteria from Chapter 7 apply to you with no special adjustment — you're the baseline the criteria were built around.
- **High Arch:** Prioritize a more cushioned, flexible sole — your foot already resists splay, so your priority is shock absorption, not containment.

Trace or tape your actual footprint below for your own records — revisit it once a year, since foot shape can shift with weight changes, pregnancy, or age.

Red Flags — When to Stop the Program and Call a Podiatrist

This book is a field manual for the everyday grind — tired, sore, overworked feet. It is not a substitute for diagnosis. If you notice any of the following, stop self-managing and get seen this week, not "eventually":

- Redness, warmth, or swelling in a toe or foot that doesn't ease with elevation and rest
- Any open sore, blister, or wound that isn't healing — especially if you have diabetes, neuropathy, or poor circulation
- Sudden, severe pain with no clear cause
- Numbness or tingling that persists well after your shift ends
- A toe or joint that looks visibly deformed, or skin that looks blue, gray, or unusually pale
- Fever accompanying foot pain or swelling
- Pain sharp enough to wake you up at night

None of the tools in this book — the Tripod Principle, the Shoe Audit, the Tactical Relief techniques — are designed to override a genuine medical problem. When in doubt, make the appointment. A same-week visit is always cheaper than a complication.

Your Foundation Log — Fillable Worksheets

The chapters gave you the tools. This section is where you actually use them. Photocopy these pages, print extras, or just write directly in the book — whatever gets you tracking consistently. A log you actually fill out beats a perfect system you never start.

The 31-Day Daily Inspection Log

From Chapter 6. Each night, run the Three-Step Scan and mark what you find. A month of data turns "my feet hurt" into a pattern you can actually act on.

Day	Temp. Check	Red-Zone Audit	Splay Test	Notes

Days 17–31, continued:

Day	Temp. Check	Red-Zone Audit	Splay Test	Notes

The Shift-Pressure Diary — A Full Quarter

From Chapters 9 and 12. Log one full week every month, or all twelve if you're building your baseline. At the end of the quarter, flip back to "The Quarterly Audit" in Chapter 12 and compare.

Week 1

Day	Surface	Intensity (1-10)	Relief Action Taken

Week 2

Day	Surface	Intensity (1-10)	Relief Action Taken

Week 3

Day	Surface	Intensity (1-10)	Relief Action Taken

Week 4

Day	Surface	Intensity (1-10)	Relief Action Taken

Week 5

Day	Surface	Intensity (1-10)	Relief Action Taken

Week 6

Day	Surface	Intensity (1-10)	Relief Action Taken

Week 7

Day	Surface	Intensity (1-10)	Relief Action Taken

Week 8

Day	Surface	Intensity (1-10)	Relief Action Taken

Week 9

Day	Surface	Intensity (1-10)	Relief Action Taken

Week 10

Day	Surface	Intensity (1-10)	Relief Action Taken

Week 11

Day	Surface	Intensity (1-10)	Relief Action Taken

Week 12

Day	Surface	Intensity (1-10)	Relief Action Taken

The 14-Day Transition Log

From Chapter 11. Track your Split-Shift → Active Hours → Full-Shift progression as you break in your new Cradle footwear.

Days 1–7 — Adaptation

Day	Hours in Cradle	Good Tired / Bad Hurt	Notes

Days 8–14 — Calibration

Day	Hours in Cradle	Good Tired / Bad Hurt	Notes

The Shoe Audit Record

From Chapter 7. Every time you consider a new pair for duty, run the Three-Minute Audit and log it here before you buy.

Date	Shoe / Brand	Splay Test	Flex-Point	Drop Test	Pass / Fail

The Quarterly Audit — Reflection

Every three months, after logging a fresh week in the Shift-Pressure Diary, answer these honestly.

What's changed in my pain levels since last quarter?

Is there a new hot spot forming?

What adjustment am I making — footwear, routine, or both?

Next quarter's focus:

Field Notes

Use this space for anything that doesn't fit in the tables — a shift that broke the pattern, a shoe that surprised you, a win worth remembering.

Glossary of Terms

- **Tripod Principle:** The three-point structural system — Heel, Big Toe Base, and Little Toe Base — that stabilizes the foot under load.
- **Coffin Shoe:** Any footwear that tapers, compresses, or elevates the foot in a way that collapses the Tripod.
- **Glass Foot:** The cumulative structural fragility that builds up after years of standing in Coffin Shoes — not a single injury, but a slow accumulation of them.
- **Cradle Footwear (Performance-Anatomical Footwear):** Wide, zero-drop, structurally supportive shoes designed to preserve the Tripod under real working conditions.
- **Splay:** The natural widening of the foot that happens when weight is placed on it — blocked by a Coffin Shoe, allowed by a Cradle shoe.
- **Micro-Break / Tactical Relief:** Brief in-shift movements — the Gravity-Dump, Calf-Pump, and Arch-Grip — that reset circulation and reawaken the Tripod without leaving the floor.
- **Shift-Pressure Diary:** The daily or weekly log tracking surface, pain intensity, and relief actions taken during a shift.
- **Good Tired vs. Bad Hurt:** The distinction between normal muscular adaptation soreness (Good Tired) and pain that signals real injury (Bad Hurt).

- **Hammer Toe:** A toe deformity in which the middle joint (the PIP joint) bends permanently upward while the tip points down.
- **PIP Joint (Proximal Interphalangeal Joint):** The middle knuckle of the toe — the site where hammer toe deformities form.
- **Corn (Clavus):** Thickened skin that forms over a bony pressure point in response to repeated friction or pressure.
- **Quarterly Audit:** The recurring three-month check-in in which you re-run the Shift-Pressure Diary for a week to catch new problems early.

More from Dr. James Whitfield

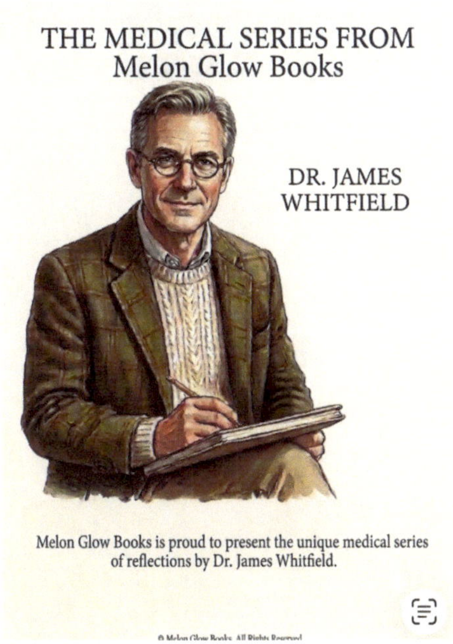

If this book helped you understand your foundation, the rest of the Whitfield library digs deeper into specific conditions and the daily maintenance that keeps working professionals on their feet:

- **The Diabetic Foot Care Handbook & Journal ("The Glass Foot"):** A comprehensive guide and daily tracking journal for patients, caregivers, and nurses managing diabetic foot health.
- **Plantar Fasciitis, Bunions, and the rest of the digital guide library:** Condition-specific, single-topic guides covering the most common complaints heard in thirty years of practice.
- **The Blood Pressure & Heart Health Journal:** A daily tracking companion for cardiovascular

health, built with the same practical, no-nonsense approach.

Visit the Dr. James Whitfield collection on Gumroad, or find the full print library at melonglowbooks.com.

The Complete Whitfield Library

Every title below is written in the same plain-English, field-manual voice — no jargon, no fluff, just what three decades of clinical practice actually taught Dr. Whitfield about keeping people on their feet.

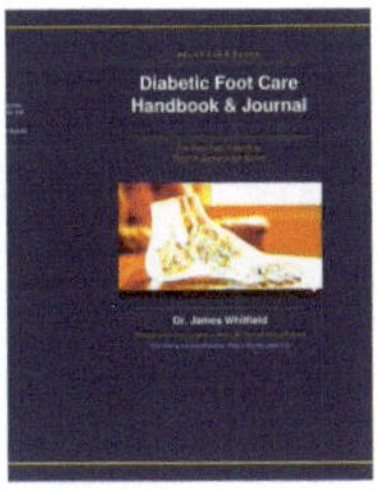

Diabetic Foot Care Handbook & Journal

"The Glass Foot": A Guide for Patients, Caregivers & Nurses

Diabetic feet are the farthest point from the heart, and the least forgiving of neglect. This handbook covers the daily inspection routine that prevents amputations, footwear and nail care done right, red flags, and a bonus chapter on gout.

Paperback: ISBN 979-8-9961392-6-2
Hardcover: ISBN 979-8-9961392-7-9

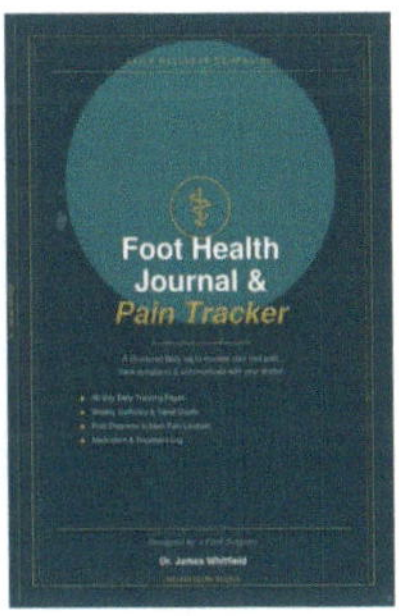

Foot Health Journal & Pain Tracker

A Daily Wellness Companion

Ninety daily tracking pages with pain scale and foot diagrams, symptom checklists, and weekly trend charts — built so you walk into your next appointment with real data instead of "it still hurts sometimes."

ISBN 979-8-9961392-1-7

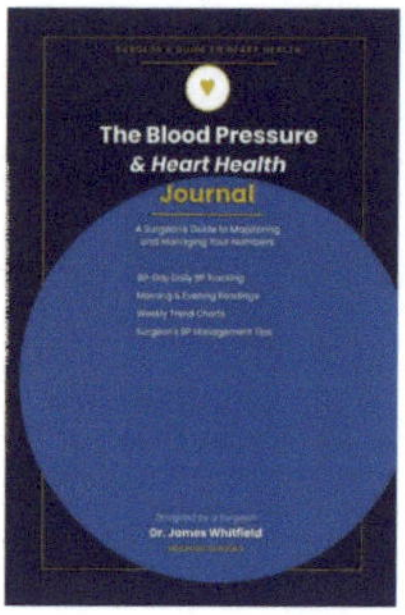

The Blood Pressure & Heart Health Journal

A Surgeon's Guide to Monitoring and Managing Your Numbers

Ninety daily log pages for morning and evening readings, vitals tracking, medication log, and thirteen weekly trend charts with a surgeon's tips on keeping the silent killer from staying silent.

ISBN 979-8-9961392-4-8

More from the Whitfield Library

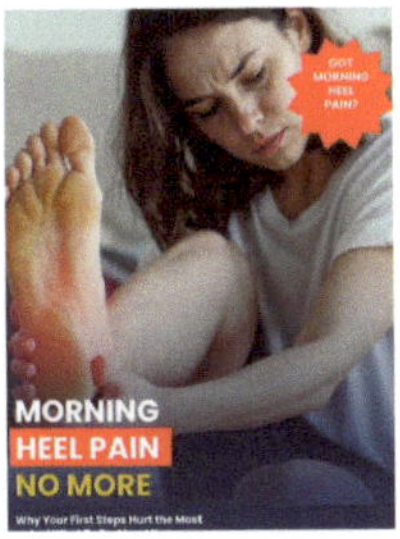

Morning Heel Pain No More

Why Your First Steps Hurt the Most

A focused, 10-minute daily routine for that first-step-out-of-bed heel pain — doctor-written, straight from three decades of practice.

ISBN 979-8-9969954-8-6

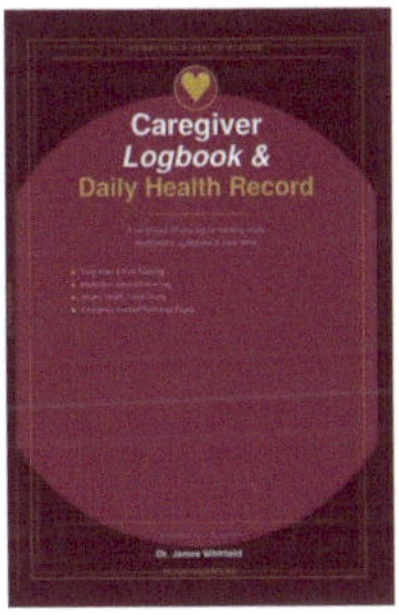

Caregiver Logbook & Daily Health Record

A 90-Day Daily Health Record

For anyone caring for a loved one: ninety daily logs for vitals, pain, mood, medications, and food, plus weekly health trend charts and an emergency contact reference page.

ISBN 979-8-9961392-3-1

Find the full print and digital library, including single-topic guides on plantar fasciitis, bunions, shoe selection, and post-surgical recovery, at melonglowbooks.com.

Also Available — Digital Guides

Instant-download PDF guides for specific conditions, all available at melonglowbooks.com:

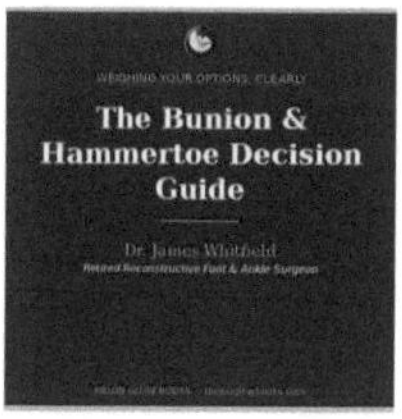

The Bunion & Hammertoe Decision Guide

Weighing Your Options, Clearly

If Chapter 5 of this book hit close to home, this guide goes deeper into exactly the decision the Wreckage Report chapter raises: when conservative care is enough, and when it's time for a real surgical conversation.

Instant PDF download · melonglowbooks.com

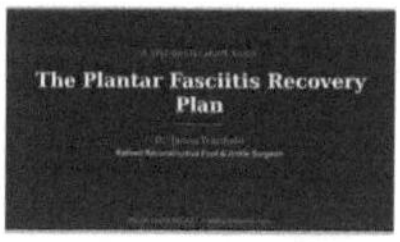

The Plantar Fasciitis Recovery Plan

A Step-by-Step Home Guide

A condition-specific recovery plan for the single most common complaint heard in thirty years of practice — that first-step-out-of-bed heel pain.

Instant PDF download · melonglowbooks.com

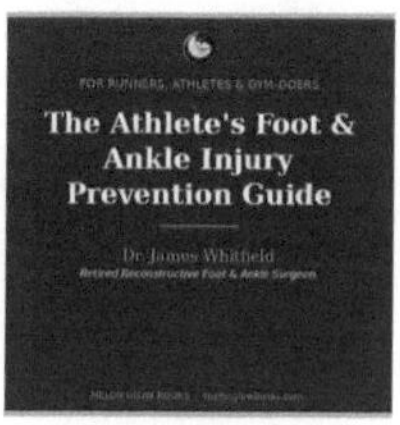

The Athlete's Foot & Ankle Injury Prevention Guide

For Runners, Athletes & Gym-Goers

Built for the active reader rather than the standing-all-shift reader — injury prevention for runners, lifters, and weekend athletes who push their feet a different way.

More Digital Guides

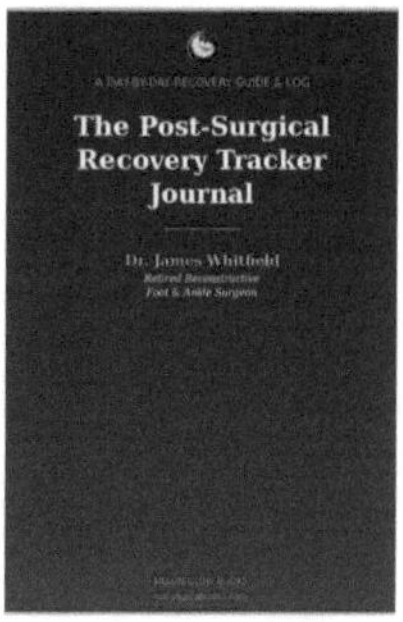

The Post-Surgical Recovery Tracker Journal

A Day-by-Day Recovery Guide & Log

For anyone recovering from foot or ankle surgery — a structured daily log to track healing, pain, and mobility milestones during recovery.

Instant PDF download · melonglowbooks.com

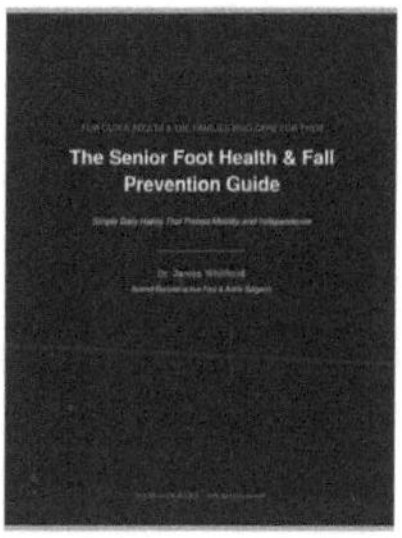

The Senior Foot Health & Fall Prevention Guide

Simple Daily Habits That Protect Mobility and Independence

Written for older adults and the family members who care for them — the foot-and-gait side of fall prevention that rarely gets discussed until after a fall happens.

Instant PDF download · melonglowbooks.com

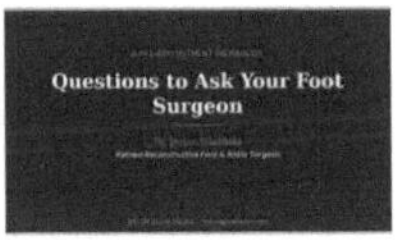

Questions to Ask Your Foot Surgeon

A Pre-Appointment Workbook

Walk into a surgical consultation with the right questions ready instead of scrambling to remember them — built from thirty years of watching patients leave appointments wishing they'd asked one more thing.

Instant PDF download · melonglowbooks.com

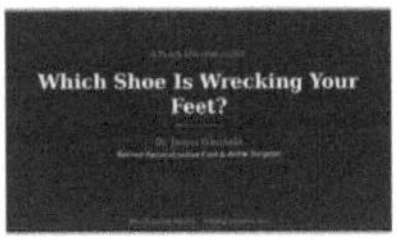

Which Shoe Is Wrecking Your Feet?

A Plain-English Guide

A practical shopping companion for spotting a Coffin Shoe before you buy it — the same Shoe Audit principles from Chapter 7, applied at the point of purchase.

Instant PDF download · melonglowbooks.com

Find the complete, current library at melonglowbooks.com.

About Dr. James Whitfield

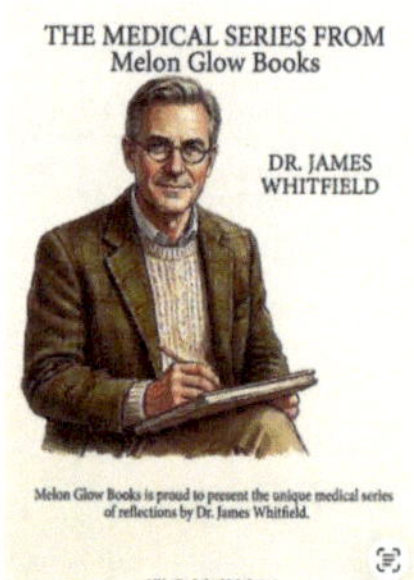

Dr. James Whitfield spent nearly thirty years practicing as a reconstructive foot and ankle surgeon, treating thousands of patients through everything from routine bunion corrections to complex diabetic limb-salvage surgery.

Now retired from clinical practice, he writes patient-education resources that distill three decades of operating-room and exam-room experience into clear, practical guidance — the kind he wishes more of his own patients had access to before their appointments.

His books and guides are written for working professionals, caregivers, and anyone tired of being told to just "power through" the pain — in plain English, without the jargon that so often stands between a patient and an actual understanding of their own body.

> *Dr. Whitfield is retired and no longer licensed to practice medicine. His books and guides are written as general educational resources, not as personalized medical advice. Always consult a currently licensed physician for diagnosis and treatment of any medical condition.*

www.ingramcontent.com/pod-product-compliance
Lightning Source LLC
LaVergne TN
LVHW051157210926
848486LV00006B/292